COPYRIGHTED MATERIAL

ARTHRITIS EXERCISES FOR SENIORS OVER 50

The prior or effective strategies and techniques for managing Arthritis through exercise

MELISSA J. LEVEY

Copyright Page

© 2024 [MELISSA J. LEVEY]

All rights reserved. No part of this book may be reproduced, stored in a retrieval system, or transmitted in any form or by any means, electronic, mechanical, photocopying, recording, or otherwise, without the prior written permission of the publisher.

This book is a work of non-fiction. Names, characters, places, and incidents are either the product of the author's imagination or are used fictitiously. Any resemblance to actual persons, living or dead, events, or locales is entirely coincidental.

Cover design by [MELISSA J. LEVEY]

Published by [MELISSA J. LEVEY]

COPYRIGHTED MATERIAL

Table of Contents:

I. Introduction

   A. Understanding Arthritis

   B. Importance of Exercise for Arthritis Management

   C. How This Guide Can Help

II. Getting Started with Arthritis Exercises

   A. Consultation with Healthcare Professional

   B. Safety Precautions and Guidelines

   C. Warm-up and Cool-down Techniques

III. Range of Motion Exercises

   A. Neck and Shoulder Mobility Exercises

   B. Arm and Wrist Mobility Exercises

   C. Back and Spine Mobility Exercises

   D. Hip and Knee Mobility Exercises

   E. Ankle and Foot Mobility Exercises

IV. Strengthening Exercises

   A. Upper Body Strength Training

  1. Dumbbell Exercises

  2. Resistance Band Exercises

 B. Lower Body Strength Training

  1. Leg Presses and Squats

  2. Wall Push-offs and Leg Raises

 C. Core Strengthening Exercises

  1. Planks and Modified Sit-ups

  2. Pelvic Tilts and Bridges

V. Flexibility Exercises

 A. Stretching for Improved Flexibility

  1. Neck and Shoulder Stretches

  2. Arm and Wrist Stretches

  3. Back and Spine Stretches

  4. Hip and Knee Stretches

  5. Ankle and Foot Stretches

 B. Yoga and Tai Chi for Arthritis Relief

VI. Balance and Stability Exercises

A. Standing Balance Exercises

   B. Chair Yoga and Tai Chi

   C. Balance Board and Stability Ball Exercises

VII. Aerobic Exercises

   A. Low-Impact Cardio Workouts

      1. Walking and Nordic Walking

      2. Swimming and Water Aerobics

   B. Cycling and Stationary Biking

   C. Elliptical Training and Rowing

VIII. Lifestyle Modifications for Arthritis Management

   A. Nutrition Tips for Joint Health

   B. Proper Hydration and Rest

   C. Stress Management Techniques

   D. Assistive Devices and Adaptive Equipment

IX. Building an Exercise Routine

   A. Creating a Personalized Exercise Plan

   B. Tracking Progress and Making Adjustments

C. Motivation and Overcoming Challenges

INTRODUCTION

Welcome to a voyage of rejuvenation and resilience, where age is just a number and movement has no limits. If you're over 50 and dealing with arthritis, know that you're not alone, and your tale is far from done. In truth, a new chapter awaits to be written—one full of life, strength, and the joy of movement.

Arthritis, with its uncomfortable grip, may have slowed you down, but it does not define you. It's only an obstacle, a roadblock on your way to recovering your enthusiasm for life. With the correct mindset and a commitment to gentle yet effective workouts, you can open up a world of possibilities and reclaim your freedom of movement.

As we begin this journey together, let us first address the elephant in the room: arthritis. Millions of people throughout the world suffer from this ailment, which causes joint stiffness, discomfort, and inflammation. But here's the thing: arthritis does not discriminate by age. It can hit anyone and at any time. However, for those of us who have reached or past the age of 50, the impact can be very strong. The good news is that arthritis does not have to be a lifelong source of pain and immobility. With the correct technique, symptoms can be effectively managed, pain reduced, and joint function improved. And this is where exercise comes in.

now I understand how the mere suggestion of exercise might elicit thoughts of anxiety or skepticism. After all, when you have arthritis, the last thing you want to do is make it worse. But here's a secret: not all exercises are equal. In reality, there are numerous arthritis-friendly activities that are expressly designed to relieve inflammation while also improving flexibility, strength, and balance.

So, let's change our perspective for a moment. Rather of perceiving exercise as a burdensome task, let us see it for what it is: a powerful instrument for regaining control of our bodies and lives. It's an opportunity to challenge arthritis's limits and rewrite our own story.

But, before we get into the specifics of arthritic exercises, let's take a moment to consider the enormous effect that movement has on our general health. The human body was intended to move; it needs and yearns for it. Movement is more than simply physical wellness; it nourishes our souls, energizes our spirits, and connects us to the world around us. Think about a period when you felt the most alive and vivid. It was most likely when you were moving—whether you were dancing freely, hiking through the countryside, or simply enjoying a leisurely stroll through the park. In those moments, arthritis was the last thing on your mind. That is the power of movement: it has the ability to transcend pain and limits, even if only for a brief moment.

Now image having that sense of freedom and vitality on a regular basis. Imagine waking up every day with a spring in your step, ready to face whatever the world throws at you. That's not a pipe dream; it's within your grasp. All it takes is a willingness to take the first step—literally—into a more active , fulfilling,   existence.

So, to my fellow arthritis warriors, I welcome you to join me on this journey of self-discovery and empowerment. We'll look at a variety of easy yet effective exercises for soothing joints, strengthening muscles, and restoring balance. Remember, this isn't a race; it's a marathon. Rome was not built in a day, nor will your mobility be recovered overnight. It will require time, patience, and perseverance. There may be days when progress feels agonizingly slow, and you will be tempted to give up. But please, don't give in to despair. Every step you take, however tiny, is a win in and of itself.

So, are you ready to begin this transformative journey? Are you ready to defy the odds, break down barriers, and reclaim your right to move with ease and grace? If so, let us take the first step together towards a brighter, more vibrant future—one arthritis-friendly workout at a time.

As we end this introduction I'd like to share a story of

courage, perseverance, and the transformational power of movement.

Sarah, a bright woman in her early sixties who, like many of us, has struggled with the hardships of arthritis. For years, Sarah let her disease control her life, submitting herself to a sedentary existence fraught with misery and resentment.

But one day, Sarah felt a flash of determination and a whisper of hope. She wouldn't let arthritis define her. Sarah set off on a voyage of self-discovery, armed with a fresh sense of purpose and moderate workouts adapted to her specific requirements.

Initially, development was slow, and doubts crept in. But Sarah persevered, pushing through the agony and celebrating each small win along the way. Her mobility and strength improved gradually with each passing day. Her joints began to relax, and the agony became more manageable.

Sarah soon found herself doing things she never imagined she could do—going for leisurely walks in the park, practicing yoga, and even dancing in her own house. With each elegant movement, she felt a surge of freedom and joy run through her veins.

But Sarah's quest did not finish there. Inspired by her own transformation, she became a source of hope for those suffering from arthritis. She spread her tale far and wide, inspiring other seniors to embrace the power of movement and restore their vitality.

And thus, my dear friends, I urge you to follow Sarah's example. Take the first step towards a brighter and more vibrant tomorrow. Accept the challenge of arthritis with courage and dedication. Remember, you are not alone on this path. Together, we can beat the odds, break down barriers, and regain our freedom to move with ease and grace.

So what are you waiting for? Let us rise to the challenge

together, striding confidently towards a life of strength, vigor, and limitless possibilities. The ability to rewrite your story is within your reach; embrace it with both hands and begin this transforming journey today.

Understanding Arthritis

Millions of individuals worldwide suffer from arthritis, which refers to over 100 distinct types of joint-related illnesses. While arthritis is generally linked with ageing, it can affect people of different ages, genders, and ethnicities. Understanding this complex ailment is critical for effectively managing its symptoms and improving overall quality of life.

1. What is arthritis?

Arthritis is defined as joint inflammation that causes pain, stiffness, swelling, and limited mobility. It can affect every joint in the body, including the hands and knees, spine, and hips. The three most frequent kinds of arthritis are **osteoarthritis, rheumatoid arthritis, and gout**.

2. Types of Arthritis:

- **Osteoarthritis (OA):** The most common type of arthritis, OA results from joint wear and tear over time. Cartilage, the protective tissue that cushions the ends of bones, eventually wears away, resulting in discomfort and stiffness.

- **Rheumatoid Arthritis (RA):** RA is an autoimmune illness in which the immune system mistakenly assaults the symposium, which is the lining of the membranes that surround the joints. This leads to inflammation, joint degeneration, and systemic symptoms including weariness and fever.

- **Gout:** Gout is caused by the development of uric acid crystals in the joints, which results in sudden and severe bouts of pain, swelling, and redness. It usually affects the big toe, but it can happen in other joints as well.

❖ ***Psoriatic Arthritis:*** Psoriatic arthritis is an inflammatory arthritis that affects people who have psoriasis, which is a persistent skin disorder. It causes joint discomfort, edema, and stiffness, which is frequently accompanied by skin sores.

3. Arthritis symptoms:

- Joint pain, which can intensify with movement or activities.

- Stiffness, especially in the morning or after prolonged inactivity.

- Inflammation and pain around the afflicted joints.

- Reduced range of motion and difficulties completing regular activities.

- Fatigue, muscular weakness, and systemic symptoms with autoimmune arthritis.

4. Risk Factors:

- ❖ ***Age***: Arthritis, particularly osteoarthritis, becomes more common as people get older.
- ❖ ***Genetics***: Certain types of arthritis, such as rheumatoid arthritis, have a genetic component.
- ❖ ***Lifestyle Factors:*** Obesity, joint injuries, recurrent joint stress, and sedentary lifestyles can all contribute to arthritis.
- ❖ ***Other Health disorders***: Certain medical disorders, such as diabetes and autoimmune diseases, may increase the likelihood of getting arthritis.

5. Diagnosis & Treatment:

Arthritis is normally diagnosed using a medical history, physical examination, imaging tests (such as X-rays and MRI scans), and laboratory tests.

The treatment goal is to alleviate symptoms, enhance joint function, and delay disease progression. Medication (such as pain relievers, anti-inflammatory, disease-modifying pharmaceuticals, and biologics), physical therapy, lifestyle changes (such as exercise and weight management), and, in severe situations, surgery (such as joint replacement) are also options.

Individuals with arthritis should collaborate closely with healthcare experts to create a personalized treatment plan that is suited to their specific requirements and goals.

6. Managed Arthritis:

- **Exercise**: Low-impact activities like walking, swimming, and tai chi can assist improve joint flexibility, strength, and overall function.

- **Healthy Lifestyle**: Maintaining a healthy diet, controlling stress, getting enough sleep, and avoiding smoking can all help with arthritis treatment.
- **Joint Protection**: Proper body mechanics, the use of assistive devices (such as braces or splints), and the avoidance of activities that worsen joint discomfort can all help protect joints from further damage.
- **Education and Support**: Learning about arthritis, joining support groups, and obtaining emotional assistance from friends, relatives, or a counselor can help people cope with their illness.

To summarize, arthritis is a complicated disorder that can significantly affect daily living. Individuals can, however, successfully traverse the challenges of arthritis and live satisfying, active lives with adequate understanding, proactive management, and support.

Remember, knowledge is power, so arm yourself with arthritis information and take control of your health and well-being.

Exercise is essential in the therapy of arthritis since it provides a slew of benefits that can help with symptoms, joint function, and general well-being.

Significance of exercise for arthritis management:

1. Jointed Flexibility and Range of Motion:

Regular exercise maintains and improves joint flexibility and range of motion. Individuals with arthritis can improve their capacity to do daily activities by engaging in modest stretching and range-of-motion exercises.

2. Strengthens Muscles Around Joints.

Strengthening exercises work the muscles surrounding the afflicted joints, giving them extra support and stability. Stronger muscles reduce joint pressure, pain, and the chance of injury or future damage.

3. Improves Joint Stability and Balance:

Balance exercises help people with arthritis improve their stability and lower their chances of falling. These exercises improve safer mobility and increased confidence in doing everyday tasks by improving proprioception (the body's knowledge of its position in space) and coordination.

4. Lowers joint pain and inflammation:

Contrary to popular assumption, exercise can help alleviate joint discomfort and inflammation linked with arthritis. Low-impact aerobic sports like walking, swimming, and cycling increase blood circulation, which supplies oxygen and nourishment to the joints while cleaning out inflammatory toxins.

5. Weight management:

Exercise is essential for weight management, especially for people who have arthritis. Excess weight adds stress to the joints, causing discomfort and inflammation. Individuals can reach and maintain a healthy weight by including regular physical activity into their daily routine, which reduces the strain on their joints.

6. Improves mood and mental health.

Exercise benefits not only the physical body, but also the mental and emotional well-being. Regular physical activity causes the release of endorphins, neurotransmitters that increase sensations of enjoyment and relaxation. Exercise can also bring a sense of success and empowerment while distracting you from your pain.

7. Increases Quality of Life:

Exercise can considerably improve the quality of life for people with arthritis by improving joint function, relieving pain, and boosting overall health. It enables people to be active and engaged in their daily lives, pursue hobbies and interests, and keep their independence and autonomy.

Finally, exercise is an essential component of arthritis care, providing numerous advantages that can improve physical, mental, and emotional health. Whether it's stretching, weight training, or cardiovascular activities, developing a well-rounded fitness regimen adapted to individual requirements and abilities is critical for effectively controlling arthritis and fostering long-term well-being.

Exercise has numerous benefits to elders with arthritis, including improved joint health, symptom relief, and overall well-being.

Common benefits of exercise for seniors with arthritis:

1. Pain Relief:

Regular exercise can help reduce arthritis-related joint pain by strengthening muscles, improving joint flexibility, and increasing the production of endorphins, the body's natural pain reliever.

2. Improved Joint Function:

Exercise preserves and improves joint function by increasing flexibility, range of motion, and stability. This enables seniors with arthritis to conduct daily activities more easily and independently.

3. Better Joint Health:

Engaging in proper activities can improve joint health by encouraging the formation of synovial fluid, which lubricates and nourishes the joints, as well as increasing circulation, which distributes important nutrients and eliminates waste products.

4. Increased Strength and Balance:

Strength training activities help seniors with arthritis gain muscle strength, which adds support to their joints and lowers their chance of falling. Balance exercises increase stability and coordination, lowering the chance of injury.

5. Weight Management:

Exercise is essential for weight management, especially for seniors who have arthritis. Maintaining a healthy weight relieves pressure on the joints, reducing pain and inflammation.

6. Boosted Mood and Mental Health:

Exercise has been demonstrated to increase mood, reduce stress, and promote general mental health. Seniors with arthritis who engage in regular physical activity frequently report lower levels of anxiety and sadness.

7. Social Engagement:

Participating in group exercise courses or activities allows seniors with arthritis to connect with others and gain support, which can boost motivation, accountability, and overall enjoyment of exercise.

8. Prevention of Co-morbidities:

Regular exercise can help prevent or treat arthritis-related co-morbidities such as cardiovascular disease, diabetes, and osteoporosis, enhancing overall health and longevity.

Nevertheless in summary, exercise is a critical component of arthritis care for seniors, providing numerous physical, mental, and social advantages. Regular exercise can help seniors with arthritis improve joint health, reduce pain, and maintain independence and quality of life.

A Comprehensive Guide to Safe and Effective Management"

First of all, there are many obstacles to overcome when dealing with arthritis, but regular exercise can help control symptoms and enhance quality of life in general. To ensure safety and efficacy, exercise must be approached cautiously and under direction. This book offers a thorough introduction to arthritic exercise, including advice from medical professionals, safety measures, and crucial warm-up and cool-down methods.

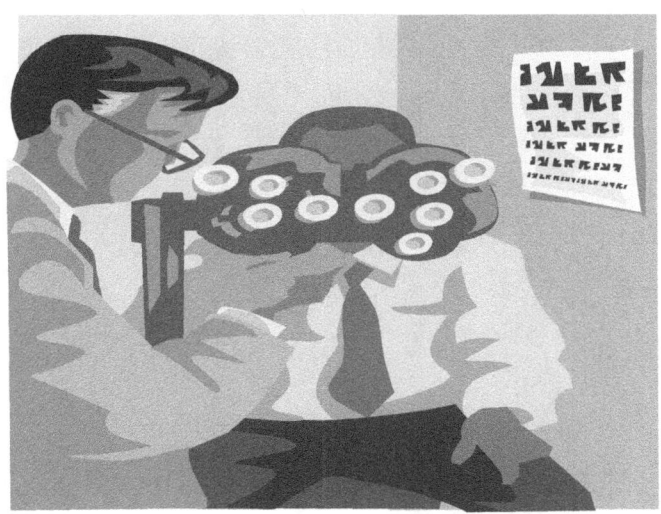

Chapter One

Talking with a Medical Professional

It's crucial to speak with a healthcare provider before starting any exercise program, especially for those who have arthritis. The significance of seeking advice from medical specialists like doctors, physical therapists, and occupational therapists is covered in this chapter. Among the subjects discussed are:

- Being aware of your particular arthritis condition: Different exercise regimens are needed for different types of arthritis. A healthcare professional's advice can help customize an exercise program to meet your unique demands.

- Medical considerations: It's critical for both safety and efficacy that you discuss any drugs, medical issues, or past injuries that may affect your exercise plan with your healthcare professional.

- Creating realistic goals: Based on your present fitness level, the severity of your arthritis, and your general health, healthcare professionals can assist you in creating attainable goals.

- Exercise recommendations: Medical specialists might suggest particular exercises, adaptations, and intensities based on your condition and goals.

Guidelines and Safety Precautions

When exercising with arthritis, safety must come first to avoid aggravating symptoms or injuring oneself. For those with arthritis, this chapter offers thorough safety measures and guidelines:

- Joint protection techniques: By using appropriate body mechanics, alignment, and technique, you can minimize pain and lower your chance of injury when exercising.

- Gradual progression: Strengthening and endurance can be achieved while reducing joint strain by gradually increasing the frequency, duration, and intensity of exercise at first.

- Pain management techniques: One of the most important things to know whether to adjust or cease a workout regimen is the distinction between "good" pain (muscle exhaustion) and "bad" pain (joint discomfort).

- Use of assistive devices: Adding braces, splints, or supportive shoes to your outfit might give you extra stability and lessen the strain on your injured joints.

- Hydration and rest: Preventing tiredness and accelerating recovery need drinking enough of water and getting enough rest in between workouts.

Methods for Warming Up and Cooling Down

Any fitness programmer must include proper warm-up and cool-down exercises, but this is especially true for people with arthritis. This chapter provides efficient warm-up and cool-down methods specifically designed with arthritis patients in mind.

- Warm-up exercises: Lightweight, low-impact activities that improve blood flow to muscles and lubricate joints, setting them up for more intense action, include walking, cycling, and range-of-motion exercises.

- Dynamic stretching: You can increase range of motion and flexibility while lowering your chance of injury by incorporating dynamic stretching exercises that replicate the movements found in your preferred activity.

- Cool-down exercises: Static stretches that target the main muscle groups should be included into your training regimen to assist avoid muscle stiffness and encourage relaxation.

- Mind-body methods: Including relaxation methods in your cool-down regimen, such as meditation, deep breathing, or mild yoga poses, can help lower stress and enhance wellbeing.

In summary:

Frequent exercise has many psychological and physical advantages and is essential for managing arthritis. People with arthritis can safely and effectively exercise to improve joint function, reduce pain, and improve overall quality of life by following the guidelines in this book, consulting with healthcare professionals, adhering to safety precautions, and incorporating appropriate warm-up and cool-down techniques.

Chapter Two

Mild Range of Motion Exercises for Alleviating Arthritis

Living with arthritis can often feel like being constrained by the limitations of inflexible joints and constrained motions. Nevertheless, integrating mild range of motion exercises into your regular regimen can provide a feeling of freedom and alleviation. This book encompasses more than just physical motions; it delves into the process of reestablishing a connection with one's body, finding the capacity for flexibility, and fostering a feeling of liberation in the face of the difficulties posed by arthritis.

Exercises for Enhancing Mobility in the Neck and Shoulders

Arthritis affecting the neck and shoulders can result in rigidity and unease, causing difficulties in performing basic actions such as rotating the head or extending the arms overhead. This chapter delves into gentle exercises specifically created to regain mobility and relieve tension in these vital regions. By engaging in these exercises, you can regain the ability to turn your head without any hesitation and lift your arms effortlessly, promoting a feeling of relief and improved mobility.

Arm and Wrist Mobility Exercises:

Arthritis affecting the arms and wrists can have a significant impact on everyday tasks such as writing, cooking, or even embracing loved ones. This chapter digs into workouts that enhance flexibility and strength in the arms and wrists, allowing you to embrace elegant movements once again. As you engage in these exercises, you'll not only experience physical improvement but also a profound sense of empowerment and delight in reclaiming control over your movements.

Back and Spine Mobility Exercises:

A stiff back and spine can greatly impede your ability to bend, twist, or stand erect with ease. Through gentle and targeted exercises, this chapter tries to release tension and restore flexibility in the back and spine, offering a pathway to emancipation from the restrictions of arthritis. As you engage in these exercises, you'll feel the weight of stiffness lift off your shoulders, replaced by a renewed sensation of freedom and lightness in your motions.

Hip and Knee Mobility

Arthritis in the hips and knees can make simple actions like walking or climbing stairs uncomfortable and complex. This chapter introduces exercises that focus on improving mobility and stability in these crucial joints, helping you to rediscover the joy of movement. As you proceed through these exercises, you'll feel the stiffness and discomfort gradually give way to a sense of emancipation and possibility, equipping you to navigate the world with greater ease and confidence.

Ankle and Foot Mobility Exercises

- Stepping into Freedom

Arthritis in the ankles and feet can make standing, walking, or even standing up from a chair tough chores. In this final chapter, we study exercises meant to promote mobility and strength in the ankles and feet, enabling you to walk into each moment with confidence and freedom. As you participate in these exercises, you'll feel the stiffness and soreness melt away, replaced by a sensation of lightness and stability that helps you to move through life with greater ease and delight.

Conclusion:

Arthritis may bring obstacles, but it doesn't have to define your existence. By embracing modest range of motion exercises with patience, compassion, and persistence, you can recapture your mobility and rediscover the joy of movement. Each stretch, each bend, and each movement is not simply a physical exercise but a journey towards greater freedom, vitality, and well-being. Embrace mobility, and allow it guide you towards a life filled with ease, grace, and possibilities.

Chapter Three

Empowering Strength

Gentle Strengthening Exercises for Arthritis Warriors"

Introduction:

Strength is not just about physical power; it's about resilience, persistence, and the unyielding spirit to overcome challenges. For individuals living with arthritis, developing strength might feel like an uphill battle, but with the appropriate exercises and mindset, it becomes a journey of empowerment. This book is a tribute to the power of strength, both physical and emotional, and includes mild yet powerful exercises to help you tap into your inner warrior and embrace your full potential.

- **Upper Body Strength Training** - Embracing Resilience

Arthritis in the upper body can weaken muscles and impair mobility, but with targeted strength training, you can restore your power and resilience. This chapter explores a range of exercises utilizing dumbbells and resistance bands, enabling you to connect with your inner strength and push beyond restrictions. As you engage in these exercises, you'll feel a sense of determination and empowerment pour over you, propelling your path towards greater strength and vitality.

- **Lower Body Strength Training** - Discovering Stability

Strong legs are the cornerstone of movement and independence, especially for persons with arthritis. In this chapter, we look into strength training routines for the lower body, including leg presses, squats, wall push-offs, and leg raises. Through these exercises, you'll not only build muscle and increase stability but also cultivate a profound sense of stability within yourself. With each repeat, you'll feel your confidence build, knowing that you have the strength to tackle any barrier that comes your way.

- **Core Strengthening Exercises** - Cultivating Inner Power

A strong core is critical for balance, posture, and total functional mobility, making it a crucial priority for those with arthritis. This chapter includes core strengthening exercises such as planks, modified sit-ups, pelvic tilts, and bridges, asking you to tap into your inner power and resilience. As you engage in these activities, you'll feel a deep connection to your center, developing a sense of stability and confidence that radiates throughout your entire body. With a strong core, you'll stand tall and meet life's problems with courage and elegance.

Conclusion:

Strength is not just about what you can lift or how far you can push yourself; it's about the inner fortitude that pulls you onward, even in the face of hardship. By accepting modest strengthening exercises with an open heart and a determined attitude, you may tap into your inner power and resilience, transforming restrictions into possibilities for progress. Each repeat, each breath, and each moment of perseverance is a testimonial to your power and fortitude as an arthritis warrior. Embrace the path, trust in your talents, and let your inner warrior shine strong.

Chapter Four

Flexibility and Freedom:

Gentle Flexibility Exercises for Arthritis Warriors"

Introduction:

Flexibility is not just about bending and stretching; it's about flexibility, resilience, and the capacity to move with ease through life's twists and turns. For persons living with arthritis, preserving flexibility is vital for managing symptoms and boosting overall well-being. This book is a celebration of flexibility, presenting gentle exercises and practices to help you accept fluidity and freedom in both body and spirit.

Stretching for Improved Flexibility - Embracing Fluidity

Stretching is a great tool for improving flexibility and alleviating stress in muscles and joints affected by arthritis. In this chapter, we explore a number of stretching exercises targeting important parts of the body, including the neck, shoulders, arms, wrists, back, spine, hips, knees, ankles, and feet. Through these simple stretches, you'll not only gain flexibility but also cultivate a sense of openness and receptivity inside yourself. Each stretch becomes an invitation to let go of tension and embrace the flow of movement, generating a deep sensation of relaxation and release.

Yoga and Tai Chi for Arthritis Relief - Nurturing Balance

Yoga and Tai Chi are ancient activities that develop flexibility, balance, and harmony between body, mind, and spirit. In this chapter, we investigate how these subtle yet effective activities might bring relief for persons living with arthritis. Through a combination of mindful movement, breath work, and meditation, you'll learn to create balance and resilience in the face of physical and mental challenges. As you flow through each yoga posture or gracefully walk through a Tai Chi sequence, you'll experience a sense of harmony and calm wash over you, nourishing a profound sense of well-being and connection to the present moment.

Conclusion:

Flexibility is not only a physical attribute; it's a state of mind and being that allows you to adapt and thrive in the face of life's uncertainties. By embracing gentle flexibility exercises with an open heart and a curious spirit, you can tap into your inner capacity for resilience and growth. Each stretch, each movement, and each moment of mindfulness becomes an opportunity to create freedom and fluidity in both body and soul. Embrace the journey, trust in your body's wisdom, and let flexibility be your guide to a life filled with grace, ease, and possibilities.

Chapter Five

Finding Stability:

Gentle Balance and Stability Exercises for Arthritis Warriors"

Introduction:

Balance and stability are the pillars upon which we build our daily lives, allowing us to navigate the world with confidence and grace. For persons living with arthritis, keeping balance and stability can be tough, but with the correct exercises and practices, it becomes an inspiring journey of self-discovery and perseverance. This book is a guide to finding stability, presenting mild yet powerful exercises to help you reclaim your equilibrium and embrace life with confidence and poise.

Standing Balance Exercises -

Standing balancing exercises are vital for strengthening stability and reducing falls, especially for persons with arthritis. In this chapter, we examine a number of exercises designed to challenge and enhance your balance while fostering a sense of stability. From simply standing on one leg to more dynamic motions like heel-to-toe walks, each exercise asks you to connect with your center and create a deep feeling of presence and awareness in every moment.

Chair Yoga and Tai Chi

Chair yoga and Tai Chi offer gentle yet effective practices for increasing balance, flexibility, and overall well-being, making them excellent for those with arthritis. In this chapter, we delve into the ideas and techniques of chair yoga and Tai Chi, providing step-by-step instructions and modifications to meet your specific needs. Whether you're gently flowing through a seated yoga sequence or gracefully moving through Tai Chi moves from the comfort of your chair, each practice becomes a voyage of self-discovery and inner harmony, nurturing balance and stability in both body and spirit.

Balance Board and Stability Ball Exercises -

Balance boards and stability balls are great instruments for increasing balance, coordination, and core strength, offering a fun and challenging approach to develop stability for those with arthritis. In this chapter, we explore a variety of exercises employing balancing boards and stability balls, ranging from easy sitting routines to more active standing exercises. As you engage in these exercises, you'll not only gain physical strength and stability but also cultivate a sense of resilience and confidence in your ability to overcome hurdles and traverse life's problems with grace and poise.

Conclusion:

Balance and stability are not merely physical traits; they're representations of our inner power and tenacity. By embracing modest balancing and stability exercises with patience, perseverance, and an open heart, you can tap into your inner capacity for equilibrium and find stability despite life's difficulties. Each workout, each breath, and each moment of awareness becomes an opportunity to restore your equilibrium and approach life with confidence, grace, and resilience. Trust in your body's knowledge, accept the journey, and let stability be your guide to a life filled with power, harmony, and joy.

Chapter Six

"Energize Your Life:

Gentle Aerobic Exercises for Arthritis Warriors"

Introduction:

Aerobic exercise is the foundation of a healthy lifestyle, providing several advantages for both the body and mind. Finding aerobic activities that are mild on the joints while still enhancing cardiovascular health can be life-changing for people with arthritis. This book can help you recapture your vitality and live a more active lifestyle despite the obstacles of arthritis.

Low-Impact Cardio Workouts:

Low-impact cardio activities are good for people with arthritis because they provide cardiovascular benefits while putting less strain on the joints. In this chapter, we look at two popular low-impact aerobic activities: walking and Nordic walking, and swimming and water aerobics. From the rhythmic motion of walking to the calming resistance of water, each exercise encourages you to embrace motion and rediscover the joy of movement. As you participate in these easy workouts, your energy levels will skyrocket, your mood will improve, and your body will come alive with vitality and strength.

Cycling and Stationary Biking—

Cycling and stationary biking are excellent ways to enhance cardiovascular fitness while reducing stress on arthritic joints. In this chapter, we will look at the benefits of cycling both outdoors and on stationary cycles. Whether you're pedaling through gorgeous landscapes or taking a virtual ride from the comfort of your own home, each revolution of the pedals represents a journey towards freedom and empowerment. As you embrace the rhythm of cycling, you'll feel the wind in your hair, the sun on your face, and the thrilling sensation of liberation that comes from moving your body with purpose and joy.

Elliptical Training and Rowing -

Elliptical training and rowing are good choices for people looking for low-impact, full-body workouts that improve cardiovascular health and muscle endurance. In this chapter, we look at the advantages of elliptical training and rowing, emphasizing their capacity to deliver a difficult yet gentle aerobic workout. Whether you're gliding beautifully on an elliptical machine or pushing through the water on a rowing ergo meter, every movement brings you closer to your fitness goals while instilling strength, resilience, and dedication. As you reach new heights with each workout, you'll realize your body's limitless potential and the endless possibilities that await you on your path to better health and vitality.

Conclusion:

Aerobic exercise is more than just getting your heart rate up; it's about living life with vitality, passion, and purpose. With an open heart and a determined spirit, you can recapture your energy, enhance your cardiovascular health, and embrace a more active and happy lifestyle despite the limitations of arthritis. Each walk, pedal, and stroke demonstrates your persistence and strength as an arthritis warrior. So lace on your shoes, get on your bike, or jump into the pool, and let the exhilarating voyage of aerobic exercise propel you to a life of health, happiness, and limitless possibilities.

Chapter Seven

Living Well with Arthritis

Lifestyle Modifications for Optimal Management"

Introduction:

Living with arthritis brings unique challenges that necessitate a comprehensive approach to treatment. While exercise is essential, lifestyle changes are also necessary for preserving joint health, managing symptoms, and increasing general well-being. This book provides a complete reference on lifestyle adjustments for arthritis management, including practical tips and strategies to help people navigate the complexity of daily living more easily and comfortably.

Nutrition Tips for Joint Health—

Individuals with arthritis benefit greatly from proper nutrition in terms of joint health, inflammatory management, and overall wellbeing. This chapter explores nutritional practices and guidelines intended to enhance joint health, including:

- **Anti-inflammatory foods:** Eating foods high in omega-3 fatty acids, antioxidants, and anti-inflammatory compounds can help reduce inflammation and relieve arthritic symptoms.

- **Balanced diet:** Eating a mix of fruits and vegetables, whole grains, lean meats, and healthy fats provides important nutrients for good joint health and overall well-being.

- **Hydration:** Proper hydration is essential for joint lubrication and flexibility. Drinking plenty of water throughout the day helps to maintain proper joint function and promotes overall wellness.

Proper Hydration and Rest—

Proper hydration and rest are critical components of arthritis treatment, encouraging joint health and general well-being. In this chapter, we examine the significance of water and rest, including:

- **Hydration strategies**: Tips for staying hydrated throughout the day, such as drinking plenty of water, eating hydrating foods, and avoiding too much coffee and alcohol.

- **Restorative sleep:** The importance of good sleep in arthritis management, as well as practical tips for enhancing sleep hygiene and fostering restful sleep.

Stress Management Techniques—

Stress can increase arthritis symptoms while also affecting general health and well-being. This chapter discusses stress management approaches to assist people cope with the challenges of arthritis, including:

- **Mindfulness and meditation**: Practices that promote mindfulness and lower stress, such as deep breathing exercises, guided meditation, and mindfulness-based stress reduction strategies.

- **Relaxation techniques**: Techniques for increasing relaxation and decreasing muscle tension, such as progressive muscle relaxation, visualization, and aromatherapy.

Assistive Devices and Adaptive Equipment:

Individuals with arthritis can benefit greatly from assistive devices and adapted equipment that increase their mobility, independence, and quality of life. This chapter examines a variety of assistive technologies and adaptable equipment, including:

- **Mobility aids:** Canes, walkers, and wheelchairs are used to improve mobility and reduce joint stress.

- **Adaptive tools**: Those are assistive equipment that makes daily chores easier, such as jar openers, ergonomic utensils, and dressing aids.

Conclusion:

Individuals with arthritis can improve their overall quality of life and manage their condition more successfully by making lifestyle changes that prioritize nutrition, hydration, rest, stress management, and the use of assistive technology. This book provides a road map for navigating the complexity of arthritis management, helping people to live well, prosper, and face life with vigor and resilience.

Chapter Eight

"Exercise Empowerment:

Building a Personalized Routine for Arthritis Management"

Introduction:

Creating an exercise plan that is personalized to your specific requirements and skills is an important step towards effectively controlling arthritis and increasing overall quality of life. This book provides a complete guide to developing a personalized workout plan, tracking progress, overcoming obstacles, and remaining motivated on your path to better health and mobility.

Creating a Personalized Exercise Plan—

Developing a personalized activity plan is the cornerstone of effective arthritis care. In this chapter, we discuss the fundamental components of building an exercise plan that meets your specific requirements and goals, including:

- Evaluating your present fitness and arthritic symptoms.
- Setting attainable goals based on your skills, preferences, and lifestyle.
- Choosing proper activities to improve strength, flexibility, cardiovascular fitness, and balance.
- Making changes and adjustments to fit any physical limits or joint pain.

By personalizing your workout plan to your unique requirements and skills, you may create the framework for a long-term and effective program that can help you manage your arthritis.

Tracking Progress and Making Adjustments—

Tracking your results and modifying your training program are critical for long-term success and continuous growth. In this chapter, we discuss ways for assessing your progress, identifying areas for development, and making required adjustments, such as:

- Keeping a workout log or using fitness monitoring apps to document your exercises, repetitions, and any changes in symptoms.

- Tracking changes in joint discomfort, stiffness, and overall mobility.

- Consult with a healthcare provider or fitness expert to adjust your exercise plan as needed based on your progress and any changes in arthritis symptoms.

Staying proactive and adaptable will ensure that your exercise regimen grows to match your changing requirements and goals, maximizing the benefits of your arthritis treatment journey.

Motivation and Overcoming Challenges:

Staying motivated and conquering obstacles are essential components of sticking to a steady fitness plan, especially when dealing with arthritis. In this chapter, we discuss ways for staying motivated and overcoming typical hurdles, such as:

- Setting small, attainable goals and enjoying your accomplishments along the way.

- Adding diversity to your fitness program to keep it interesting and engaging.

- Seeking help from friends, family, or support groups to keep you accountable and motivated.

- Developing coping methods for dealing with pain, exhaustion, and other issues that may emerge during exercise.

By building a positive mindset and resilience, you can overcome hurdles and remain devoted to your exercise regimen, empowering yourself to make long-term changes in your arthritis treatment journey.

Conclusion:

Creating a personalized fitness plan can help you manage arthritis while also improving your general health and mobility. You may empower yourself to take control of your arthritis management journey and live a more active and satisfying life by developing a personalized plan, measuring your progress, keeping motivated, and conquering obstacles. This book provides a road map for negotiating the intricacies of developing an exercise program, allowing you to accept exercise as an essential component of your arthritis care plan.

In closing this voyage through our arthritis exercise book, I am reminded of the profound impact that small, consistent efforts can have on our lives. As we come to the end of these pages, I urge you to reflect not only on the exercises you've learned but also on the journey you've undertaken.

Arthritis isn't just a condition, it's a daily battle that can affect every aspect of our existence. But through dedication and perseverance, we have the power to redefine our relationship with arthritis and reclaim control over our bodies.

I'm reminded of Mrs. Judith, a woman who once struggled to perform even the simplest duties due to the pain and stiffness in her joints. She felt confined in a body that no longer felt like her own. However, with the guidance of this exercise book, Sarah began to implement gentle movements into her daily routine.

At first, progress was sluggish, and there were moments of frustration and doubt. But she persisted, deriving strength from the knowledge that each stretch and exercise was a step towards reclaiming her life. Gradually, she observed improvements - increased flexibility, reduced pain, and a renewed sense of vitality.

But perhaps the most significant transformation was internal. Mrs. Judith found herself approaching each day with a newfound sense of hope and optimism. She no longer felt defined by her condition but empowered by her capacity to overcome it.

And so, as we bid farewell to these pages, let us carry forward the lessons learned and the fortitude gained. Let us remember that while arthritis may be a part of our narrative, it does not have to be the defining phase.

With determination, resilience, and the power of movement, we can continue to write a life filled with pleasure, vitality, and endless possibilities.

Thank you for embarking on this journey with us. May your path ahead be filled with health, happiness, and the freedom to live your life to the utmost

www.ingramcontent.com/pod-product-compliance
Lightning Source LLC
Chambersburg PA
CBHW070411230526
45471CB00006B/2760